Essential Oils for Natural Healing

Ultimate Recipes for Balance, Beauty, Home, Personal Care & Wellness

ABIGAIL BRADLEY

Legal & Disclaimer

The information contained in this book and its contents is not designed to replace or take the place of any form of medical or professional advice; and is not meant to replace the need for independent medical, financial, legal or other professional advice or services, as may be required. The content and information in this book has been provided for educational and entertainment purposes only.

The content and information contained in this book has been compiled from sources deemed reliable, and it is accurate to the best of the Author's knowledge, information and belief. However, the Author cannot guarantee its accuracy and validity and cannot be held liable for any errors and/or omissions. Further, changes are periodically made to this book as and when needed. Where appropriate and/or necessary, you must consult a professional (including but not limited to your doctor, attorney, financial advisor or such other professional advisor) before using any of the suggested remedies, techniques, or information in this book.

Upon using the contents and information contained in this book, you agree to hold harmless the Author from and against any damages, costs, and expenses, including any legal fees potentially resulting

Table of Contents

Introduction

For years aromatherapy oils have been a part of human civilization. The early ancestors found ways to use and harness their amazing capabilities and since then became known as one of the most safe and effective ways to provide natural healing in our lives. One of the most notable uses of essential oils is its capability to relieve stress.

In this world where everything is fast and people are always moving, it's no wonder that stress became a part of their everyday lives. No matter how hard you try, this cannot be avoided. Stress is present in all facets of your life. From work, studies and family, even with your relationship – stress is always present. However, there are ways to relieve stress and one of the most effective ways as mentioned is with the use of essential oils.

Congratulations and thank you for purchasing this book about essential Oils. Inside you will learn and discover the ways on how to use essential oils effectively for everyday use, what are the types of essential oils that are effective for you, how to prepare them, and a whole lot more.

So start right now and discover the power of these essential oils. Not only will it be useful to relieve your stress but you will also discover its other potential and eventually use them. Enjoy learning and start using them!

Chapter 1 – The Science of Aromatherapy

Our mind is a master controller of sorts that governs how each and every system in our body functions. As such, providing the right mood to one's mind greatly affects the overall function of the entire body. Each of our senses provide the mind so much stimulus that massages, hearing soothing music, and seeing lush greens and calm sceneries have the ability give out positive energy, so does being exposed to certain fragrances enhance our bodily functions. This is what we call "Aromatherapy".

Aromatherapy is a practice of using aromatic substances to simulate the body and produce favorable mental states. Since ancient times it has been used to soothe illnesses, improve creativity and even sexual drive. The practice uses essential oils that are either applied and massaged into the skin or heated in a diffuser to release their fragrances. Flowers, leaves, roots and barks of plants, and sometimes even the sap of trees are extracted to produce these fine oils.

Benefits of Aromatherapy

Some may argue about the benefits of aromatherapy, but it has been widely tested to provide a significant improvement in minimizing anxiety, and improving overall comfort levels of people that have recurring health conditions. It targets mainly the minds current state, stimulating positive thoughts and thereby alleviating pain. It has been known to even decrease the pain felt from needle insertion by patients undergoing dialysis, and some minor surgeries that require full consciousness and only small doses of anesthesia.

To bring out the safest, purest, best effects of Aromatherapy, it is essential to use natural ingredients as much as possible. Since these oils have more benefits than just being aromatic, they can also be used as a substitute for chemical based substances, thereby almost eliminating one's dependence on them.

Whether using it as a deodorizer, natural wood polisher, or even as a substitute to most toiletries and beauty care materials like shampoo, soap, and even toothpaste, it is sure to be safe as it is effective.

A Focus On Essential Oils

The use of Essential Oils has been around even during the time of Ancient Egypt, and has been famous as a luxury item, valued in the lines of gold and precious stones. Our ancestors have found out that the essences of certain plants (herbs, shrubs, or even trees) can be preserved indefinitely through meticulous extraction of their oils, and storing it on darkened and sealed vessels so increase its shelf life even further.

However, the term "Essential Oil" itself came from an abbreviated form of "Quintessential Oils". This is a concept from ancient Greece, pertaining to the states of matter. According to this, matter is composed of the 4 basic elements (fire, water, air and earth and spirit). Certain combinations of these bring about everything we see today. The method of extracting quintessential oils is akin to viewing it as a form of preserving the "life essence" of a certain plant.

Crude concepts were used back in the day to capture these essences, and as technologies improve, so does the method and efficiency of these extractions. Nowadays distillation, using steam or through high-tech machinery provides consumers with purer essences, with increased yield volumes. The ISO or the International Organization for Standardization oversee also certifies that manufacturers produce these substances through strict standardized ways.

.

Chapter 2 – Common Types of Essential Oils

Common Types of Essential Oils

Essential oils contain rich amount of potent antioxidants which purify, beautify, and heal. These properties are significant reasons why they are popularly used as premium ingredients of perfumes, soaps, hair products, and skin care. Their powerful therapeutic benefits make them vital part of many medicinal products and aromatherapy. Each of them contains unique healing powers that can help restore, treat or enhance health condition. It is important to check their therapeutic use and how to use them for maximum benefits.

Bergamot

Bergamot is known for its citrusy, orange with a hint of sweet floral scent. It comes from Bergamot trees which thrive in Ivory Coast, Italy, and in other countries in Southeast Asia. Its oil extract comes from peels which are cold-pressed or steam distilled. Bergamot contains active "bergaptene" chemical component that increases the sensitivity of skin to sunlight. This sensitizing, high phototoxic constituent of Bergamot is usually distilled to avoid adverse effect to users. However, distillation does not give a hundred percent guarantee and the danger remains. Better take precaution when using this essential oil by avoiding long exposure to sun's UV rays.

Bergamot's aroma makes it one of the best ingredients of deodorizer and vaporizer. Most colognes, lotions and perfumes have this oil. It is also used in incense. Others use the oil as flavor to their tea beverages. It is an excellent oil choice for bath, massage and aromatherapy. When used in aromatherapy, it fights depression, uplifts moods, inspires positive attitude and boosts confidence. Bergamot is helpful during periods of grief, anxiety, and sadness.

Bergamot is an antidepressant, sedative, disinfectant, spasmodic, analgesic, digestive, and febrifuge. It treats anorexia disorder, stress, anxiety, and depression. The potent components of this essential oil stimulate spleen, liver as well as regulate digestive system. It combats oily skin as well as cures acne, boils, cystitis, abscesses, psoriasis, cold sores, eczema, itching, and halitosis. For precautionary measures, dilute Bergamot essential oil before skin topical application because it can burn skin.

Cedarwood

Cedarwood has woody, balsamic aroma which enhances the feeling of centeredness and strengthens inner peace. It is best to use when you are under emotional stress and powerlessness. It is calming, grounding and stimulating. This oil is used in embalming purposes during early Egyptian period. Its aroma is sweet, woody and reminiscent of mothballs.

Cedarwood essential oil is known to cure acne, coughing, dandruff, cystitis, arthritis, stress, and wounds. It fights spasms, increases urination, removes toxins, salt, fats, and excess water from the body. It regulates women's monthly menstrual cycle, kills insects, prevents inflammation, balances nervous disturbances and stops fungal growth.

When used in aromatherapy, Cedarwood essential oil promotes calming effect which eliminates stress and uplifts the spirits. It is also known to be the best oil to treat skin issues, respiratory problems and urinary tract infection.

Chamomile

Chamomile essential oil is an extract from Chamomile leaves and is steam distilled. It blends perfectly with other essential oils. It is used as ingredient of creams, lotions and beauty products. It is a strong antibiotic, anti-depressant, antiseptic and stress-reliever. To release tensions, it is best to use it in vapor or steam therapy.

Chamomile oil can cure spasms, prevents infections, stops biotic growth, fights depression, uplifts moods, protects wounds, reduces vessels swelling and soothes fever inflammation. It is also used to improve nervous system condition, digestion and liver function. It removes gas, assists in proper bile discharge, regulates obstructed menstruation and kills bacteria.

Eucalyptus

Eucalyptus is considered the best topical essential oil that is used in salves and liniments. It comes from the tree of Eucalyptus which is found in Australia. The oil is extracted from twigs and leaves through steam distillation process. It possesses powerful, distinct aroma which enhances good mental concentration.

Eucalyptus essential oil contains "cineole" which gives its healing properties that include antiseptic, diuretic, antispasmodic, stimulant and decongestant. Its cooling property fights fevers and migraines as well as muscles pains. It is also used in deodorizers. It is also used to treat bronchitis, cold sores, flue, sinusitis, catarrh, diabetes, intestinal germs and mental fatigue.

Jasmine

Jasmine essential oil is an extract which originated from China. It is obtained through solvent extraction which produces solid substance. Then it will undergo the process of placing flowers on top of fats to get the fragrance. It takes days before the essential oil becomes usable.

It one of the most expensive and powerful oils that effectively heals many diseases and emotional disturbances. It has calming and relaxing properties. It eases childbirth as well as emotional depression. Jasmine essential oil also helps eliminate addiction, enhance libido, promotes respiratory health and alleviates stress.

It also prevents scars, protects wounds from infection, reduces spasms, relieves cough, regulates menstrual cycles and increases breast milk production.

Lavender

Lavender is another popular essential oil. Its extract comes from flowers, buds and leaves of lavender plant through steam distillation process. Its name comes from "lavera", a Latin term which means "to wash". True to its name, lavender is known as effective stress-reliever, antibacterial, antifungal, diuretic, decongestant, inflammatory, sedative and deodorizer. It treats migraine problems, flu and common colds. It is safe to treat scrapes, wounds and minor cuts among children. Its medicinal benefits treats asthma, allergies, chicken pox, dermatitis, athlete's foot, acne, colic, dysmenorrhea, cystitis, hypertension, earache, headache, flatulence, insect bites, labor pains, rheumatism, sores, migraine, scars, stretch marks, scabies, whooping cough, vertigo and oily skin. It also cures respiratory disorders, nervous system problems, indigestion, immune system issues, insomnia, blood circulation abnormality and normalizes urine flow.

Lavender oil has great scent that soothes and relaxes during therapeutic practices such as aromatherapy or massage sessions. Adding few drops to your bath water or pillows before sleep stimulates calmness and relaxation. It heals broken spirits, normalizes moods and balances emotions. It is popularly used for colognes, perfumes, lotions, salves, oil baths, toilet water and room sprays. It mixes well with other essential oils and gives off sweet, floral aroma.

Peppermint

Peppermint is an intense and concentrated form of essential distilled oil. When undiluted, it can make sinuses tingle. It exudes fresh, minty and sweet aroma when diluted. It contains menthol which brings cooling sensation as well as eases muscle pains and tension headaches. It is proven to be a potent aphrodisiac.

Peppermint oil in aromatherapy helps in rejuvenating body, mind and spirit. It can be blended with other essential oils to promote stamina, alertness and health. Its cooling properties enhance moods, fight irritation, help in mental focus, aid digestion and eliminate congestion symptoms.

Peppermint has many uses such as pain reliever, expectorant, anesthetic, analgesic, antispasmodic, astringent, hepatic, carminative, stomachic and decongestant. It is usually used to reduce flow of milk and abnormal discharge, relax muscle spasms, stops hair loss, rejuvenates skin, protects against sepsis, strengthen gums and removes gas. It is best in asthma, flu, headache, scabies, vertigo, sinusitis, colic and exhaustion.

Peppermint also stimulates memory and brain health, stops hemorrhage, firms up muscles, clears congestion, assists in bile discharge, and eases difficulty in breathing. It assists in relieving obstructed menstruation, promotes perspiration, reduces fever, expels off catarrh and phlegm.

Sandalwood

Sandalwood gives off woody scent. This essential oil comes from mature tree wood chips which are extracted and distilled to its purest form. It is used as ingredient of lotions, massage oils, incense, creams, aftershaves, facial care products, mouthwash, and vaporizers. Its balsamic, sweet and woody scent improves as it aged.

It offers many therapeutic benefits in aromatherapy like alleviating chest pains, relaxing agent to relieve stress, helping urinary tract mucous membranes to function well and calming nerves. It is also known to stimulate sex because of its aphrodisiac property. It is anti-inflammatory and hydrates the skin. Sandalwood is used for spiritual cleansing, chakra purifying and emotional purging.

Sandalwood is an exotic and expensive essential oil. Its scent lasts long and assists senses to focus clearly. It soothes fever inflammation, protects cuts or wounds from danger of infection, firms muscles, tightens gums, clears spasms and prevents continuous hair loss. It is commonly used to heal scars, relieves flatulence, increase urine flow, keeps skin healthy and smooth. Sandalwood is proven good in reducing the danger of hemorrhage, cures common colds and cough, stimulates sharp memory, boosts immune system, soothes nerves and helps in reducing high blood pressure. It alleviates bronchitis, dry skin, oily skin, chapped skin, laryngitis and leucorrhea.

Tea Tree

Tea Tree is discovered by James Cook, a famous explorer in Australia. It was widely used by indigenous inhabitants of the land for many medicinal and therapeutic purposes. Its spicy, warm aroma is often used in aftershaves, creams and colognes.

For aromatherapy, it promotes purifying, rejuvenating and cleansing effects. It boosts immune system and stimulates systemic functions of the body. It is used to stop bacteria and other viral infections, protects wounds to avoid sepsis, promotes nutrients absorption, hastens scars healing and cures coughs.

It is one of the most favorite essential oils with so many uses. It is known to heal skin blemishes as well as improves the health of the scalp to promote hair growth. It is a good cure for athlete's foot, dandruff and burns.

Chapter 3 – Choosing The Right Essential Oils

Essential oils are therapeutic and wellness products that help improve your health and well-being. This is the reason why you should be careful in choosing the right essential oils. Every scent and flavor gives off a different result depending on the status of your condition and its reaction to your body. When choosing essential oils, it is best to consider the quality.

Importance of Choosing the Right Essential Oils

Just because you saw a shelf full of essential oils in groceries or drugstores, it does not mean that you're going to get anything that you see. These oils heal you from pain, illnesses, and stress. That is why you need to consider some things before buying the oils that you need.

Not Just an Oil: Looking for Quality

Contrary to what others say, these essential oils are not just the generic ones seen in your nearby drugstore. They contain ingredients that are therapeutic and holistic to the body. That is why you must get oils for their quality and not for what you see.

Buy oils from reputable establishments or companies.

Many companies out there claim they offer oils of superior quality. However, in truth, they are just telling that to sell their products. In choosing the right essential oil company, you have to make sure they adhere to the following: purity, price, quality, service, and reputation. There are times when the price is high, yet the quality is superior that you won't think twice of buying them. We advise that you get a company that has great customer service and is always there to help you when something goes wrong with their product. Overall, research the companies that you think are good and see if they have positive feedbacks and a good reputation in the industry.

Research about the oil.

Also, to know more about the company, you need to research about the oil you plan to buy. Do you think it is perfect for treating your back pain or curing your cough? Look at its ingredients and check for reviews to see if they are as effective as they claim to be. There are stores and companies that offer samples---take advantage of that and test it on your skin or body before buying the real thing. This way, you will know if it works well or if you develop allergic reactions. Researching won't take a lot of time. What is important is you think of your health first.

Train your own nose and know more about the varieties.

As said above, you don't just get any oil you see in groceries. You have to determine the scents and variants of essential oils to find out their uses.

If you need to calm down from stress, depression, and anxiety, picks the lavender oil. To help you relax, buy chamomile, ylang-ylang, or clary sage. For a long day at work, choose rosemary or peppermint to awaken the senses and keep you energized. The variants are endless---you just have to research about them to see what works best for you.

How the plants are grown.

This is part of your research, as you will need to see how the plants are grown. It is actually better to get organic oils because they don't have harmful chemicals. Buy essential oils that are provided by local growers, as they are well taken care of and have higher quality.

How the oils is distilled.

The best essential oils are the ones best processed and retains their therapeutic value. There is no additional pressure or heat, making the oils pure and clean. What you get is the oil itself and the great results they give.

Thinking About Your Safety

Always keep your safety in mind when choosing essential oils. You don't want to endanger your body just because you heard this kind of oil is great or that the scent is good. Below is a guide on how to know that what you are buying is safe.

A lot of turnover.

Buy from a source that has a quick turnover time. Most, if not some, of the ingredients have their own expiration dates. For example, citrus goes stale easily, as it has the shortest shelf life. Make sure the oils you buy are also stored well and are not exposed much to heat or direct light. There are also some variants that need to be refrigerated, like butter. Just make sure that you don't get essential oils that are expired and stale.

Pure and safe.

These oils should not contain harmful chemicals that can endanger your health. They must be pure; thus, it is always good to buy samples first and try if they are good to your body. Also, make it a habit to look at the information at the back of the bottle.

Linked to trusted memberships and companies.

Established suppliers provide data and test results that say their essential oils are safe to use. This is their way of showing transparency and telling people that they are willing to answer any questions. Another way to prove credibility is being members with trusted associations, such as National Association for Holistic Aromatherapy (NAHA). This means they abide by NAHA's ethics standards and regulations. Another possible indicator of ethical and therapeutic standards is having trained aromatherapists to look at their oils.

All in all, it is a must to be safe in picking the right essential oils by looking at their quality. By using the guide above, you can get oils that will not only treat your ailments, but also keep your body safe.

Chapter 4 – Essential Oil Applications

Essential Oils for Everyone

There are people who are skeptical in the wonders of essential oils, believing they are not for everyone. They also assume that these oils are not practical to use and are hard to apply. People still doubt its wonders and prefer not to use them even when they need it. What they do not know is that these oils are for everyone and there are different ways to apply them.

Choosing an Application Method

Each and every oil has its own desired effect, so it's a must to know what you are looking for. Applying essential oils depends on your condition or ailment, as well as the prescription of your doctor. It is possible that other oils have better results when rubbed on the skin, while there are those that work well when inhaled. If you do not know what application works best for you, let us be your guide on that. Below is some useful information that tells about the different application methods.

Direct Inhalation

These oils can be inhaled directly using different methods and techniques. Inhaling them can help address mode effects and respiratory ailments.

Dry Evaporation

Place some drops of your desired essential oil either on a cotton or tissue. Allow the oil scent to evaporate in the air for a few seconds to one minute. Once you think the smell has settled, you can either sniff it or leave it anywhere in the room. Sniffing the scent directly gives you a more intense dose, while living it within your area gives a milder exposure to the oil scent. The latter also helps treat the ailments of other people by just naturally inhaling it.

Spray

Deodorize a room or set a mood in a meeting by using essential oils in spray form. Just place several drops in a bottle containing the solution, shake it, and spray in the air. This is perfect when you plan to have the whole family during the holidays or are hanging out with friends. Give your room a positive vibe by spraying citrus or pine oils. Peppermint oils, on the other hand, stimulate alertness.

Topical Application

Topical application of essential oils is one of the most common methods among children and adults. They are usually done on wounds, bruises, or the need for skin relief. However, please note that you need to dilute the oil in different ingredients before applying it on your skin because it is very strong and potent. Dilution depends on the type of application and the person who needs to use it.

Rub or Massage

Once you have diluted the oil, apply it on the affected area through gentle rubbing. Put about 1 to 2 drops of oil on your palm and massage the area in a circular motion. Repeat the massage a few times until you feel relief. This type of topical application is commonly used among adults. However, make sure to read the directions the essential oil bottle for application.

Bath

Have a relaxing bath by using essential oils. Add a few drops of the oil in bath water and wait for it settle down before stepping in. By using this method, you get the best of both worlds because the skin absorbs the oil and, at the same time, you inhale its scent. However, some other oils might be too sensitive to the skin, so it is best to disperse them. One of the things that can disperse these oils is bath salts. If you want a relaxing bath, you can also mix two cups of Epsom salt, one cup baking soda, and three cups of sea salt. Then add seven to eight drops of your desired oil, specifically lavender oil, before entering.

Compress or dressing

We believe this method should be done when the doctor has prescribed it. Once the oil is mixed thoroughly, you can apply it either directly on the area which is affected or by using a cloth or cotton ball. Another technique is mixing the oil with water. Soak a cloth in the solution and place it on the sore muscle or affected area. Using essential oils in compress and dressing gives better results if there is hot or cold water.

Gargle

Do this when you have diluted the essential oil with water. Mix them together, gargle it, then spit it. Never swallow it. Oil that is perfect for gargling is tea tree oil. Even a few drops the oil in a glass bottle filled with water will give you much comfort.

Aerial Diffusion

Aerial diffusion works best if the essential oils are placed in a device with water. Together with heat, this application method disperses the oils so their scents fill a room or area with natural fragrance. By doing so, you set the mood for everyone. You can create your own diffuser or buy one in any store.

Steam

Before anything else, please note that this method is not recommended for children younger than 7 years old. Add several drops of essential oils in a bowl of steaming water, which will help quickly vaporize the oil. Then, place a towel over your head and on the bowl. Breathe deeply. Unlike dry evaporation, this inhalation procedure is very direct and potent because you are in contact with the strong scent. It is important to close your eyes when inhaling the oil, so they won't sting. One example is the eucalyptus oil. This is perfect for those who have respiratory ailments and colds because the oil can slowly smoothen the breathing and clear lungs or nose.

Candle

Light a normal or soy candle and burn it for about five minutes. Extinguish the fire and place one drop of essential oil on the melted wax. Light the candle again and make the fragrance of the oil fill the room. Be careful in doing this because essential oils are flammable.

Indeed, essential oils are for everyone because they can be applied in different ways. You just have to find the right method depending on your preferences and needs. Let our guide above help you find the method that suits you well. However, if you are not sure which method to use, consult a trusted aromatherapist.

Chapter 5 – Making Your Own Essential Oil

Computerized and programmed methods are not the only ways essential oils are made. There are also multiple "primitive" means of extracting or distilling oil out of any plant material.

The only downside is that the heat used in these native ways of distilling or extracting can lessen a little amount of the purity of the essential oil you are making. However, take note of the "little". It's doesn't matter whether your essential oil is *absolutely* pure or not. The important thing is it's still guaranteed to give you great results as to whatever purpose your own-produce essential oil may have.

There are six methods introduced and it's up to you to choose which approach is comfortable for you. So here are the different ways on making your own essential oil:

First Method

Note first that the essential oil produced in this method is NOT suitable for consumption.

1. For two weeks, immerse the plant material inside a rubbing alcohol container (with cap on).
2. After the said time frame, gently transfer it out into a wide container and wait for the alcohol to evaporate.
3. Now collect the left oil in the wide container.
4. Store in dark glass container.
5. This will last for about six months.

Second Method

1. Grab a small bottle and put ½ teaspoon of white vinegar, ½ cup of olive oil (or grape seed, jojoba or almond), and 1 tablespoon of ground up plant material.

2. For three weeks, place this bottle in a windowsill where it's warm and exposed to sunlight.
3. Shake the bottle twice a day (every 12 hours) continuously for the entire time frame.
4. You can now gather the liquid by straining with unbleached cheese cloth.
5. Store the essential oil in a dark, glass container.
6. Don't forget to label.
7. This essential oil will last for up to six months.

Third Method

You might like this method because it can be prepared pretty quickly.

1. Get 2 cups of olive oil (or grape seed, jojoba or almond) and stir with ½ ounce of your chosen plant material.
2. For about six hours, cook the mixture in a crock pot on low heat.
3. Strain; just like the previous method, use unbleached cheese cloth in this step.
4. Store the essential oil in a dark, glass container.
5. Label if deemed necessarily.
6. The oil will last for up to six months.

Fourth Method

1. Using olive oil (or grape seed, jojoba or almond), half-fill a large glass bottle.
2. For the remaining half volume, put as much plant material into the bottle.
3. Cap or cover the bottle.
4. For 24 hours, let it sit in a dark place with cool temperature.
5. After the said time frame, shake the bottle very well.
6. Let it sit again for three more days.

7. Now strain the mixture using cheese cloth.
8. Store the essential oil in a dark, glass container.
9. Note: if the scent is not strong enough, repeat the process but this time, add more plant material.
10. This essential oil will last for up to six months.

Fifth Method

1. Put a ground up plant material in linen or cotton bag.
2. Tie it tightly and put in a pot filled with distilled water.
3. Boil the water and slowly simmer for about 24 hours.
4. You should see the oil on the water surface.
5. You may have to squeeze the bag and get the oil off the water surface.
6. Store in a dark, glass container.
7. Cover the container with a thin cloth.
8. Let the oil sit for a week. This will allow extra water to evaporate, leaving pure essential oil behind.
9. This will last for up to a year.

Sixth Method

This is the best method in making essential oil.

1. Get a crock pot and fill with distilled water.
2. Place the plant material.
3. For 24 hours, cook on low heat.
4. After which open the crock pot and leave it that way for about a week.
5. Get the oil away from the water surface.
6. Store in a dark, glass container.
7. Cover the container with a thin cloth.
8. Leave it for another week to allow extra water to fully evaporate, leaving only essential oil behind.
9. This essential oil will last for up to 12 months.

Dos And Don'ts In Aromatherapy

DO: It is okay to utilize a bottle with a rubber dropper top as containers for your essential oils. However, this is only applicable to essential oils combined with carrier oils at low dilution for a few months.

DON'T: A follow up to what is stated above; it means you can't store undiluted, pure essential oils in a bottle with a dropper top. This is because the rubber will become mush, consequently ruining the oil.

DO: As mentioned multiple times, always store your oils in a dark glass; cobalt blue or amber will do. Along with that, you must always keep your bottles (containing oils) in a cool and dark place. This is an important method in preserving the significance and effectiveness of whatever oil you may have in store in those containers.

DON'T: Do not use unclean bottle. Make sure the bottles you are using are purely clean and absolutely dry.

DO: To have no problems transferring multiple bottles from place to place, you can put your bottles in wooden hinged boxes. There are available wooden boxes at craft stores so you won't have a problem finding one. You can also use wooden floppy disk holders or anything that fits the role.

DON'T: Do not miss even a single step and adhere appropriate time frame. Follow all instructions above carefully.

Now you're ready to for the next stage – preparing your own recipes!

Chapter 6 – Essential Oil Recipes

Now that you know how to make essential oils out of any plant material, it's time to get to the real deal! In this chapter, I will introduce a lot of essential oil recipes classified into different aspects. As you may already know, there are so many essential oil recipes and each of them has their own corresponding purpose. But here, you will get to know the most important recipes with the most useful applications.

Home (Natural Cleaning, Home Purification & Etc)

Carpet Deodorizer

Ingredients:

- 1 16 ounce box of baking soda
- 20 drops of Lavender
- 10 drops Lemon

Procedure:

Get a large bowl and mix the essential oils and the baking soda. Ensure that you're able to mix them thoroughly because soda can be a little sticky. Mixing well also prevents the lemon oil from staining your carpet (since basically it's colored yellow). You can also your favorite essential oil as add-ons if you want it.

After mixing, store in an airtight container or in a glass jar. If you want to recycle, you can use an old spice container (the one that has holes in it). That way you can simply "shake" the deodorizer onto the carpet. You can also use powder sifter containers perfect for carpet deodorizers and body powders.

To use:

Simply sprinkle the deodorizer onto the carpet you want you to clean. Allow the deodorizer to sit for about 15 – 20 minutes. Now start vacuuming on the same carpet.

Fabric Softener Recipe

Ever want to make a simple fabric conditioner? Well, this recipe only needs a single ingredient to make it work. And that ingredient is vinegar.

To use:

During the rinse, add ½ cup of vinegar to your laundry as substitute for a commercial fabric softener.

Note:

Your eyebrows may have met once you read the word "vinegar" above. Don't be surprised though. Vinegar may have an abrasive smell but it's actually anti-viral and anti-bacterial. What makes vinegar more interesting is it eliminates soap residues on your clothing and it could soften clothes when used during rinse. Above all, it's very cheap.

Don't worry, your clothes won't smell as long as you don't pour excessive amount of vinegar.

Air Freshener

Everybody would dream for an aromatic home. Consider this mist air freshener recipe to give your home a fresher air.

Ingredients

- 30 – 40 drops of your favorite essential oil (blend samples below)

- 4 oz. spray bottle (don't use bottles that previously have cleaning content like hair products)
- 1.5 fl. ounces of high-proof alcohol and 1.5 fl. ounces of hydrosol or distilled water

Sample essential oil blends

Blend no.1

- 14 drops Bergamot
- 20 drops Lime
- 2 drops Rose
- 4 drops Ylang-ylang

Blend no. 2

- 6 drops Lavender
- 9 drops Lemon
- 15 drops Clary Sage

Blend no. 3

- 8 drops Grapefruit
- 20 drops Rosemary
- 2 drops Spearmint
- 4 drops Peppermint

Blend no. 4

- 15 drops Spearmint
- 15 drops Bergamot

How to prepare

1. Fill your spray bottle with 1.5 fl. ounces of alcohol and 1.5 fl. ounces of distilled water.
2. Add 30-40 drops of the essential oil blend of your choice.

3. You can try for only 20 drops of essential oil depending on your aromatic sense or if you consider a household member who is sensitive to smell.
4. Note that you should not fill the entire bottle to leave room for shaking the mixture well.

Bed Linen Spray

Take care of your bed linen with this recipe.

Ingredients:

- 30-40 drops of a relaxing or calming essential oil (blend samples below)
- 4 oz. clean spray bottle; it must have a setting of fine mist. Avoid using bottles that previously have hair or cleaning products.
- 1.5 fl. ounces of high proof alcohol and 1.5 fl. ounces of distilled water

Blend samples of relaxing or calming essential oils

Blend no. 1

- 10 drops Bergamot or Mandarin
- 10 drops Clary Sage
- 10 drops Lavender

Blend no. 2

- 15 drops Bergamot
- 20 drops Roman Chamomile (do not use German chamomile because it has weak properties)

Blend no. 3

- 30 drops Roman Chamomile (do not use German chamomile for the same reason above)

Blend no. 4

- 15 drops Bergamot or Grapefruit
- 15 drops Sandalwood
- 2 drops Jasmine
- 2 drops Rose

Blend no. 5

- 2 drops Jasmine
- 10 drops Sandalwood
- 3 drops ginger
- 2 drops Ylang-ylang
- 3 drops Lime
- 10 drops Bergamot

How to prepare

1. Fill your spray bottle with 1.5 fl. ounces of alcohol and 1.5 fl. ounces of distilled water.
2. Now fill 30 to 40 drops of the blend of your choice.
3. Do not make it full so you can shake the bottle before each use.

Dryer Sheet Recipe

Make your laundry naturally fragrant in a gentle way by using this essential oil dryer sheet recipe. You can also enjoy cost savings against using commercial dryer sheets.

Ingredients:

- 5 drops essential oil (any of your favorite as long as it has thin viscosity and pale colored)

- Scraps of white or natural cotton fabric approximately 5" x 5". Do not use colored fabrics.

How to use:

1. Pour 1 – 4 drops of your favorite essential oil into your chosen cotton fabric.
2. Now dry your clothes as you normally do, but this time, include this cotton fabric in the dryer.
3. Once done, your clothes will have the fragrance of your favorite essential oil.

For Wellness (Weight Loss, Energy, Physical Wellness & Etc)

Improved Energy Recipe

Use any of the set of ingredients and blend them to energize your body and mind whenever you feel fatigue. This helps in stimulating vitality right when you need it.

Set no.1:

- 2 drops Ginger
- 2 drops Grapefruit

Set no.2:

- 2 drops Grapefruit
- 1 drop Cypress
- 2 drops Basil

Set no.3:

- 2 drops Lemon
- 1 drop Frankincense
- 2 drops Peppermint

Set no.4:

- 3 drops Bergamot
- 2 drops Rosemary

Diffuser blend:

1. Produce about 20 drops of your chosen blend by multiplying any set by 4.
2. Put these oils in a dark glass and roll the bottle between your hands as a way of mixing them.
3. Refer to the manufacturer's instructions and add the right number of drops from your own blend to the diffuser.

Ease Fear Recipe

Blend no. 2 (when you need to be energized)

- 2 drops Bergamot
- 3 drops Grapefruit

Blend no. 3

- 1 drop Clary Sage
- 2 drops Frankincense
- 2 drops Jasmine

For diffuser blend

1. Select one of the blends above (preferably no. 1) and multiply amount by 4 because you need to achieve 20 drops.
2. In a dark colored glass bottle, add the oils and roll bottle between your palms.
3. Add the right number of drops (according to manufacturer's instructions) to blend to the diffuser.

Massage Oil Recipe

Ingredients:

- 10 – 12 drops of Sore Muscles Blend
- 1 fl. ounce carrier oil (like Sweet Almond Oil)

Sore Muscles Blend:

- 1 drop Black Pepper
- 2 drops Ginger
- 5 drops Eucalyptus
- 4 drops Peppermint

How to prepare:

1. Get a dark, airtight glass container.
2. Pour in the ingredients and mix well.
3. You can double or triple the recipe.

How to use:

1. Apply about ½ - 1 teaspoon to affected areas and massage.

Versatile Energy Recipe

This recipe is considered versatile because you can use it in multiple ways: as massage oil, for bath, and for footbath.

Ingredients:

- 1 drop Cinnamon
- 2 drops Peppermint or Eucalyptus
- 5 drops Lemon

For bath:

Combine all ingredients and simply add to teaspoons to your water-filled bath tub.

For footbath:

Combine all ingredients and simply add 1 teaspoon to your foot bowl.

For massage oil:

1. Your carrier oil must be unrefined, virgin cold pressed, and pure.
2. Dilute with 2 ounces almond, grape seed, or vegetable oil.

Weight Loss Blend

When you inhale this blend, the microscopic molecules will travel all the way to your hypothalamus where the satiety center is located; this is responsible for your fullness or hunger feelings.

When the molecules reaches this part of your brain, the satiety center will be 'tricked' that you are already 'full' releasing signals to rest of your brain, including your stomach, telling you that you are 'full'. The next time you eat, you will feel full sooner!

Ingredients:

- 1 drop Ylang-ylang
- 4 drops Lemon
- 30 drops Grapefruit
- 1 teaspoon coarse sea salt

How to prepare:

1. Get a handy aromatherapy inhaler. It must be PET plastic bottle or a dark glass.
2. Now pour 1 teaspoon of course sea salt.

3. Add the remaining ingredients.
4. Shake

How to use:

1. You can use this recipe to suppress your appetite and curb your cravings by inhaling it for about 5 minutes (or refer to step 4 and 5).
2. Use your inhaler every time you crave for a lot of food.
3. You can carry it in your bag or anywhere as long as it's handy.
4. Take three slow, deep, and long breaths from the aroma.
5. Take a little break and repeat step 4 again for 3 times.
6. Make sure your nose is flooded with the aroma and scent to make this blend more effective.
7. Use this every time a nice food triggers your appetite or before eating.

For Balance (Emotional Wellness, Mood & Serenity)

Relax and Calming Recipe

Ingredients:

- 5 drops of Lavender
- 7 drops of Roman Chamomile
- 1 fl. Ounce carrier oil (like sweet almond)

For foot massage:

Combine all the oils and put in dark, glass container. Make sure the bottle is clean and air-tight. This relaxing oil will surely delight you with its calming effect. All you have to do is to massage gently into the feet of the person who needs more calm and relaxations. Note that a strong sedative effect can be brought by the Roman

Chamomile so it's not recommended for you to do tasks that require concentration (like driving, studying, etc.).

Diffuser blend:

When you plan to create a diffuser blend, the blend must have a ratio of 1 drop of Lavender to 2 Drops of Roman Chamomile and add to your diffuser.

Anti-Anxiety Recipe

You would be glad to hear you can make an effective anti-anxiety recipe on your own. There are four blends of recipes available; feel free to choose any of the set of ingredients.

Set no.1:

- 2 drops Bergamot
- 3 drops Sandalwood

Set no.2:

- 1 drop Frankincense
- 2 drops Clary Sage
- 2 drops Bergamot

Set no.3:

- 1 drop Lavender
- 1 drop Rose
- 1 drop Vetiver
- 2 drops Mandarin

Setno.4:

- 2 drops Clary Sage
- 3 drops Lavender

For diffuser blend:

Obtain a total of 20 drops of your chosen blend by multiplying any of the set of ingredients above by 4. Put the oils in a dark, glass bottle. Roll the bottle between your hands as a way of mixing them. Now add certain number of drops (depending on the manufacturer's instructions) from your own blend to your diffuser.

Gratitude Essential Oil

Ingredients:

- 10 drops Grapefruit
- 20 drops Bergamot
- 10 drops Frankincense
- 10 drops Cypress
- 2 drops Ginger
- 5 drops Ylang-ylang

How to prepare:

- Mix all the ingredients in a glass bottle (make sure it's clean)
- When you meditate, pray, or give thanks, diffuse as you would other essential oil
- You can also experiment your own "celebration blend"

Confidence Recipe

Ever wanted to increase your confidence? Try this recipe to boost your self-esteem.

Blend no. 1

- 2 drops Rosemary
- 3 drops Orange

Blend no. 2

- 3 drops Bergamot
- 2 drops Bay Laurel

Blend no. 3

- 2 drops Cypress
- 3 drops Grapefruit

Blend no. 4

- 1 drop Jasmine
- 4 drops Bergamot

For diffuser blend:

1. Choose one of the blends and multiply the quantity by 4 to achieve 20 drops.
2. In a dark colored glass bottle, put your chosen blend and roll the bottle between your palms.
3. Add this to your diffuser; make sure you follow the manufacturer's instructions.

Happiness Recipe

These blends will help uplift your mood and put you in the positive vibes.

Blend no. 1

- 2 drops Orange
- 2 drops Frankincense
- 1 drop Geranium

Blend no. 2

- 1 drop Grapefruit
- 1 drop Ylang-ylang

- 3 drops Bergamot

For diffuser blend:

1. Select one blend and multiply quantity by 4 to have 20 drops.
2. Put them in a dark colored glass.
3. Refer to the manufacturer's instructions of your diffuser and add the right number of drops.

For Beauty (Hair & Scent)

Scented Hair Recipe

Ingredient:

- 1 drop of Sandalwood, Lavender, or Rosemary

How to use:

1. Select one from the options above and gently drop to your hairbrush's bristles.
2. Brush your hair well.
3. The essential oil will leave a nice aroma to your hair.

Bath Oil Recipe

Essential oils that are safe to your skin can be dropped directly to your bathwater but it's much better to use bath oils because concentrated essential oils have the tendency to settle on one spot and not mix with water.

Ingredients:

- 20 drops Lavender
- 2 fl. ounces carrier oil (like Jojoba)

How to Use:

1. In a glass bottle, blend the oils together.
2. You can also double or triple the recipe for more use.

Men's Cologne Recipe

Ingredients:

- 1 fl. oz. Distilled water
- 2.5 fl. oz. Perfumer's Alcohol or High Proof Vodka
- 15 drops Patchouli
- 15 drops Mandarin or Bergamot
- 3 drops Ginger or Black Pepper
- 5 drops Bay Laurel
- 2 drops Neroli oil
- 3 drops Vetiver or 5 drops Oakmoss Absolute

How to Prepare

1. Sterilize a 4 oz. bottle. (it's good to have a sprayer on top)
2. Put water and alcohol
3. Mix in the oils
4. Shake well
5. Let the cologne sit for several days
6. Every day, you must shake the bottle twice
7. Do this until you feel like the oil has blended and mellowed out, thus ready for first use

How to Use

1. Shake the bottle well
2. Apply a considerable amount to an area inside your forearm
3. Continue usage if it doesn't irritate

For Personal Care (Ailment Treatments, All-Around Relief & Etc)

Arthritis Aromatherapy recipe

There are two sets of blends and you only need to choose one.

Set no. 1:

- 10 drops Helichrysum
- 10 drops Roman Chamomile
- 2 fl. ounces Carrier oil

Set no. 2:

- 4 drops Black Pepper
- 20 drops Roman chamomile
- 2 fl. ounces Carrier oil

Note:

Use carrier oils that contain anti-inflammatory properties such as Pomegranate Seed, Jojoba, emu oil, and Hemp Seed oil. Emu oil also has robust anti-inflammatory properties though it's not a vegetable oil.

To Use:

Choose one set and blend all these oils well. Store the blend in a dark and air-tight glass container.

Using small amount of oil, smoothly massage it into arthritic joints and neighboring areas. But before that, it is important to visit your doctor and ask him about proper massage techniques suitable for your specific form of arthritis. There are also cases wherein the doctor may prohibit any massage.

Once you feel discomfort in your arthritic joints, stop using and visit your doctor as soon as you can.

Aromatherapy for Menstrual Cramps

This one is simple. Menstrual cramps can make women quite uncomfortable but this aromatherapy recipe has got the right solution.

Ingredients:

- 5 drops Peppermint Essential Oil
- 1 fl. Ounce Jojoba
- 3 drops Lavender Essential Oil
- 4 drops Cypress Essential Oil

To use:

Combine all ingredients in a dark glass bottle.

Smoothly massage a small amount into the affected areas, particularly the abdominal part.

Congestion Aromatherapy Recipe

Ingredients:

- 4 drops Peppermint Essential Oil
- 26 drops Ravensara Essential Oil
- 30 drops Eucalyptus Essential Oil
- Cotton Ball or Aromatherapy Inhaler

To use:

Mix all the ingredients in dark glass bottle. It is suggested to use a bottle with a built-in dropper insert (orifice reducer).

When using cotton balls, apply 2-3 drops into the cotton ball and hold the cotton ball near to your nose and gently inhale occasionally; do not inhale excessively.

When using aromatherapy inhaler, immerse the orifice reducer into the oil blend then insert into the tube and close the cover (or cap). Hold the inhaler near to your nose and gently inhale.

Grief Coping / Relieving Recipe

This recipe will help you in times of grief.

Blend no. 1:

- 3 drops Cypress
- 2 drops Rose

Blend no. 2:

- 3 drops Sandalwood
- 2 drops Rose

Blend no. 3:

- 3 drops Sandalwood
- 1 drop Rose
- 1 drop Neroli

For diffuser blend:

1. Select one blend.
2. Multiply the ingredients by 4 to achieve 20 drops.
3. Blend in a glass bottle that is colored dark and roll between your palms to mix.
4. Refer to the diffuser's instructions and add the right number of drops.

Insecurity Coping / Relief Recipe

This is like a follow-up to the confidence recipe but this blend focuses more on alleviating feelings of insecurity, consequently relieving you from it.

Blend no. 1:

- 1 drop Frankincense
- 2 drops Bergamot
- 2 drops Cedarwood

Blend no. 2:

- 1 drop Vetiver
- 1 drop Jasmine
- 3 drops Bergamot

For diffuser blend

1. Select one blend and multiply the quantity by 4 to obtain 20 drops.
2. Put in a bottle with dark colored glass then roll bottle between your hands as a way of mixing.
3. See the diffuser instructions and add the right number of drops.

Now you've been introduced to these exciting recipes, it's time to put them into good use! What's left for you to do is to incorporate what you have learned and try the recipes in real life. Every single recipe may come in handy when you need them.

Conclusion

You have reached the end of the book. I hope that you have learned so much from this reading journey and be able to do your essential oils on your own. All you need is a little creativity and spending a little of your time to make this new and chemical free products. What's more, you might be able to make it as a hobby and eventually earn from it, right?

Stress has been one of the most common problems people are facing nowadays. Having learned other ways to relieve stress is a great benefit. Aside from discovering other ways to alleviate stress through the use of these essential oils, you are also helping the environment, hence promoting a clean and green living. With the prominence of hazardous chemicals in the market, everyone wants to live healthy and of course be safe. So like I said, I hope this book will be an instrument for you to keep on using this alternative way in keeping yourself stress free. Continue taking care of your body, and yes, share them with your friends and family members too. You might be surprised that one day, you can create your own brand of homemade stress relief essential oil that is unique and could potentially be a new innovation in the market. How's that for an added benefit?

Again, congratulations for purchasing this book and if you enjoyed it, please take the time to share your thoughts and post a review on Amazon. It'd be greatly appreciated!

Have fun and enjoy the benefit of these essential oils!

-- Abigail Bradley

www.ingramcontent.com/pod-product-compliance
Lightning Source LLC
Chambersburg PA
CBHW071138280526
45787CB00003B/1321